How to Correct High Blood Pressure Without Medications

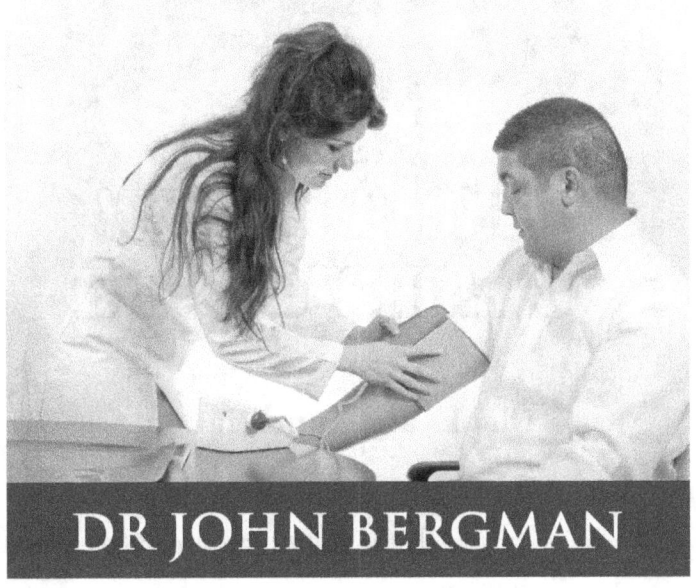

DR JOHN BERGMAN

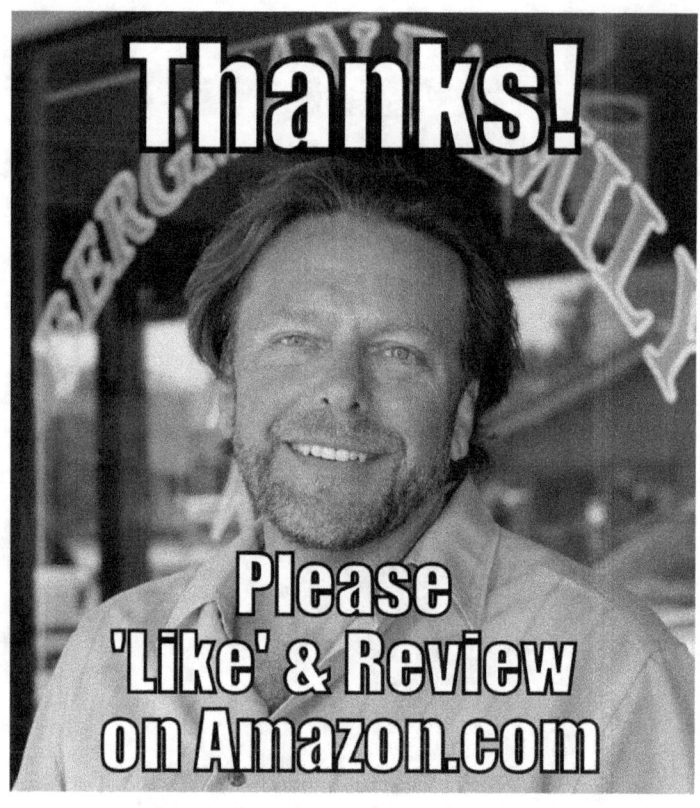

Thanks and Appreciation

I need to thank my patients for having the courage to stand up to a medical system that is not just broken but dangerous. It takes an incredible amount of courage to take responsibility for your own health. Too many people today abdicate authority over their health to a medical professional, submitting to medical procedures blindly and many times with disastrous results.

I have always approached health issues with the idea that the human body is intelligent and there are reasons for its responses to environmental stimulus (that is what doctors and people call symptoms). If you look at all symptoms whether it is High Blood Pressure, Depression, Reflux, even Cancer has intelligent responses by the body to deficiencies or toxicities then the solution for those symptoms or conditions will be so clear. This driving thought has been inspiring me to research the true source of disease and the solutions of those diseases.

I am going to include real patients with real problems that have been mistreated by an obsolete medical system. I have changed the names of the patients but their ages and the symptoms and the therapies they endured are real. I want you to appreciate the true courage to take charge and responsibility for one's health and to go against the health authorities of today. Throughout history, to change a broken system has taken vision, courage, and a focus on a different idea. Imagine when Galileo first had the idea that the earth wasn't the center of the universe. He was threatened with excommunication from the church ridiculed by most of those in power. His idea's were proven true and he is today hailed as a hero. The people who take charge of their own health are my heroes and this book is dedicated to that independent spirit and vision. God Bless You Folks.

John Bergman D.C.

About the Author

I was raised in Burbank, California, the youngest of four children and the only boy. Being raised by a single mom with three sisters was amazing. I was taught self reliance and was raised with incredible freedom. My mom and sisters were loving and nurturing and I could hardly wait to get away from that. Looking back on those times my family gave me the strength and confidence to explore on my own. My dad was in my life only for a brief time, I remember him as kind, wise and loving and as good a dad as he knew how to be. As soon as I could, I took a test to get out of high school at 16 years old I moved away from home and right into college at 17 year old. I changed my major at school every time I got interested in something new, I loved learning. This passion for learning has been with me my whole life, it has driven me to completely different worlds. I dropped out of college at 20 years old because I wanted to start a family and I met an older woman who was amazing (I was 17 and she was 19). To pay for college I worked the summers in construction saved like crazy and lived very cheaply. A box of mac-n-cheese was a good dinner at 25 cents. I built my first home at 21, had my first son by 25 and divorced by 27. I focused in on the family and home but I neglected my wife. That was a hard lesson. My next lesson: I felt stagnant in my life. I needed a change so I prayed to God for a change. God listened …I was hit by a car breaking both of my legs, fracturing my sternum and skull, bruising my heart and liver. There is an old Chinese curse "may you get what you wish for". Well I got the change in my life that I prayed for and it was, and has been, amazing. Being obsessed with learning I now had to learn how the body healed. It is interesting that one of my last jobs was to install an x-ray room for a Chiropractor, Dr. Anthony. Little did I know that doctor would be adjusting me in a wheel chair just weeks after I finished his x-ray system. Dr. Anthony inspired me on the body's ability to heal. I also had a team of medical doctors, that were brilliant in saving my life, they were lacking in my belief that my body would heal completely. They knew drugs and surgery, I needed more. I started Chiropractic college, limping in pain but hopeful in an innate intelligence that Dr. Anthony told me about. He said my body was designed by God and health was its natural state. I liked that belief system. It turned out that I had a real gift for anatomy, I just knew how things worked. I felt I found my calling. I was born to be a Chiropractor and teacher. After graduation I taught human dissection, anatomy and several technique courses. When I started practice I put my new knowledge of how the body was designed to heal and I saw miracles. I saw high blood pressure normalize, fibroids just go away, ear infections vanish, joint pain that was there for years just go away. My patient would ask me questions and if I didn't know the answer I would look it up so my knowledge base grew. I started holding regular classes on every health subject you could imaging. I started my health classes just teaching basic anatomy, because I thought that if everyone knew how their body worked they would be amazed and really appreciate how wonderful they were. I started to video tape these classes and people were asking for books I have written so here is my next book on how to correct high blood pressure.

Contents

Disclaimer

You must not rely on the information in this book and/or video series as an alternative to medical advice from your doctor or other professional healthcare provider. If you have any specific questions about any medical matter, you should consult your doctor or other professional healthcare provider.

If you think you may be suffering from any medical condition, you should seek immediate medical attention. You should never delay seeking medical advice, disregard medical advice, or discontinue medical treatment because of information in this book and/or video series.

Any change in medication, diet, and/or exercise should be directed by a qualified health care professional.

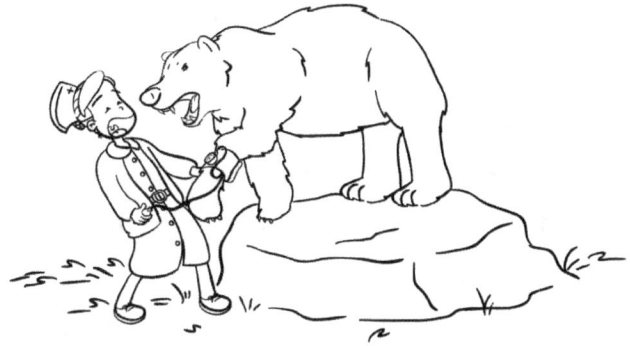

High Blood Pressure is NOT a Disease

There has never been a species on this planet that couldn't
self regulate their functions. By functions I mean regulation
of: digestion, blood pressure, blood sugar, cholesterol,
hormone levels, etc… There is no beaver with high
cholesterol, no bear with high blood pressure, and no diabetic
deer. There are certain laws like the law of gravity that
pertain to biology. All the species on this planet (humans fall
into that category) have to take in nutrients, eliminate waste
products, regulate an immune system, reproduce, and self
repair. Any species that can't perform these basic functions
would not survive. Any species that requires medications to

perform these basic functions is a sick species. To use a medicine to alter physiology has become accepted by our society. We are being programmed by the media that medications are not just good for you, you need the drugs to be healthy and happy. Picture the commercial of the person suffering from depression then they get the medication and they are happy running through the field of flowers. The narrator rattles off the myriad of effects hoping you keep your ears closed to the side effects and your eyes on the happy field of flowers.

For an example of a sick species that will not survive imagine if a giant herd of elk had; 30% of their population had diabetes, 50% had cancer, 30% had high blood pressure and 30% had pre-hypertension (almost high blood pressure). Would we be sending doctors and drugs to help the herd or would we want to find out why the herd was sick. Those are the numbers of America today 30% of Americans have diabetes, 50% have cancer, 30% have high blood pressure and 30% had pre-hypertension (almost high blood pressure). So either being American is bad for your health or we are doing something wrong with life style and/or health care that is causing our population to one of the sickest the world has ever known.

This book is a guide to how your body regulates blood pressure. Too many people today are rushed thru a medical system that is broken. Today's medical system is based on a flawed paradigm of symptom = drug philosophy. People today are diagnosed and drugged without being educated on the "why" behind their condition or disease. Our current health care system lacks respect for the natural body's regulatory system. Over-riding your natural blood pressure regulation with medications is a violation of biologic law. By chemically altering physiology with a medication and not respecting that the human species is self regulating and self healing, this approach can lead to other diseases and ill health. High Blood Pressure is NOT a disease it is a clue to how your body is working. Your blood pressure goes up and down for a huge number of reasons, circumstances and conditions. People can take medications that can lower blood pressure however does this lead to a healthier longer life? Or does lowering blood pressure with a medication lead to other diseases? To answer these questions look at the effects of the medications...also called side effects. The list below is a **partial list** of effects from medications given to lower blood pressure:

- Asthma symptoms

- Cold hands and feet

- Depression

- Erection problems

- Insomnia and sleep problems

- Dizziness

- Headache

- Irregular or very rapid heartbeat (palpitations)

- Swollen ankles

- Anemia

- Constipation

- Drowsiness

- Dry mouth

- Fever

- Diarrhea

- Heartburn

- Excessive hair growth

- Fluid retention

- Headaches

- Joint aches and pains

- Swelling around the eyes

- Stuffy nose

Case # 1 Ella a 24 year old single mom with 2 kids, who was 30lbs over weight comes to me with chronic headaches, high blood pressure, high cholesterol, insomnia, and mild depression. She was prescribed 2 drugs for blood pressure, 1 for cholesterol, 1 for sleep, and 2 for the headaches. She had no energy and complained to her medical doctor, he would just compliment her on her "perfect blood pressure and cholesterol levels". Too many times patients are not heard by their doctors. I was lucky enough to have a brilliant mentor Dr. William Jacobson who said "to find out what is wrong with people you have to do 2 things. 1. Ask them, and 2. Listen" now that sounds easy but to really hear someone takes skill.

I actually talked to Ella we did an exam and x-rays I found out that she had had those headaches since she was a teenager. I took an x-ray of her and found she injured her neck years earlier when she was in gymnastics and it had been missed and never corrected. Her care began immediately, her headaches went away within a week, without the pain her blood pressure normalized without the medications, and with less pain her cholesterol also normalized and her sleep patterns changed all within a month. Being drug free and pain free, her energy skyrocketed and her health returned. (NOTE) : Ella within 6 months lost 25lbs and has her kids on a health based lifestyle which includes healthy eating and regular nervous system check-ups.

How to Diagnose High Blood Pressure

To officially be diagnosed with high blood pressure your blood pressure has to be taken on 3 different occasions at 3 different times of the day over a 2 week span. These protocols are rarely done in today's medical system. The reason for taking this time to make the correct diagnosis is that the drugs used for decreasing high blood pressure can have disastrous effects on the body. That is why the 2 week protocol. It is better to err on the side of caution then to rush someone to a diagnosis and drugs they don't need. In working with high blood pressure patients for nearly 15 years, I have never had any patient tell me that the correct 2 week protocols were followed. They are rushed to be diagnosed and drugged without being educated on the "why" behind their condition or disease. When a blood pressure medication or any other medication is prescribed your health is vitally dependent on the quality of questions you ask your doctor. Like: "why did my blood pressure read high on your machine?", "How long do I have to take this medication?" or "What are all of the effects of this medication and do the negative effects increase the longer I take this drug?" "Will these medications give me a longer better quality of life?"

This book will give you a strong base into how your body works and help you ask those vital questions to give you a healthier longer more vital life.

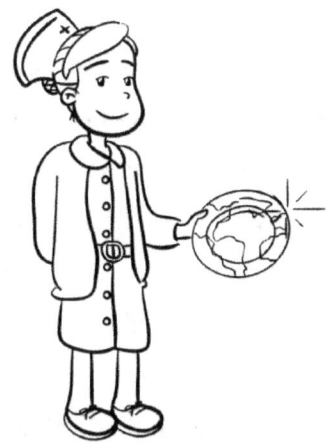

Flat Earth Medical Technology

**"Doctors are men who prescribe medicines of which they
know little, to cure diseases of which they know less, in
human beings of whom they know nothing"**

   Voltaire 1692-1788

Most of the doctors in this country are bound to treatment
protocols dictated by the medical groups they work with or
the organizations they belong to. Those treatment protocols
are usually called "standards of care". Currently most of the
standards of care of the American medical community,
dictate that when vital signs, like blood pressure and heart
rate are taken, if there is a blood pressure number higher than

the very narrow range that you are compared with, you are labeled or diagnosed normal or pre hypertension or hypertension.Those standards of care are taught in medical school, which drills into the young Doctors a symptom = drug mantra. This symptom= drug approach leaves little respect for the natural regulatory processes that occur in the body. The majority of the medical doctors take a pharmacological approach first with some diet advice given possibly. I have a number of medical doctors as patients. When I ask them if they consider the total effects of multiple medications on a person's physiology. They consistently express frustration in that the patients just don't change their life styles to lower blood pressure or lower cholesterol or blood sugar, so they feel they need to give the medications to change the blood pressure, cholesterol, etc… So there is this focus in the medical system that everyone is supposed to have the same range of blood pressure. No matter the age or physical health of the person. In reality there is a huge difference in the health of a person who has a naturally regulated blood pressure of 120/80 compared to a person who is taking a medication to force their blood pressure artificially to 120/80. You must remember the blood pressure number is analytic not diagnostic or it is a snap shot in time to what the body is adapting to at that moment the blood pressure number is NOT diagnostic of a disease. A huge problem in today's medical world is the blood pressure number used to diagnose and also is a basis for treatments usually drugs or pharmaceutical intervention. In addition, the medical doctors of today have little training in nutrition or the cause of disease and little to no training in the appreciation of health as the natural state of the body. The medical system of today is focused on disease and the treatment of disease, not on health and the methods of restoring and regaining health. It is like a financial analyst who only studies poverty giving investment advice.

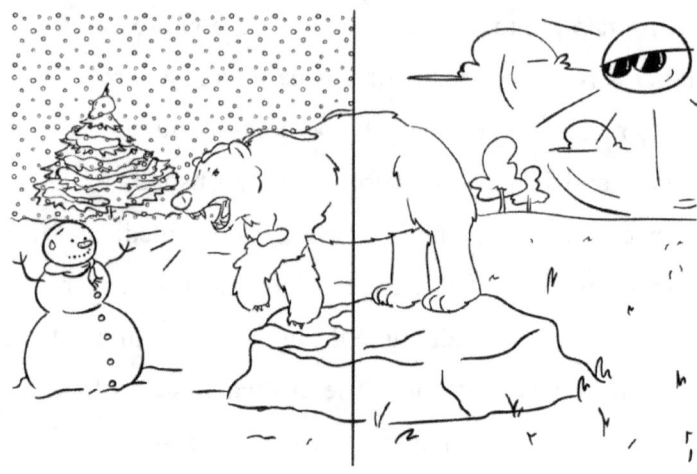

Symptoms: Disease or Adaptation?

With only a few minutes between patients the doctors have to hold to those "standards of care" protocols, so aspirin, blood pressure drugs cholesterol drugs and pain relievers are passed out without the doctor or patient ever asking the vital questions "why" are my blood pressure/heart rate or cholesterol numbers off or why is the body giving these symptoms. And these drugs can have disastrous results. Take for example a "baby aspirin" oh boy what marketing genius came up with calling the 4th deadliest drug in America (aspirin) "Baby aspirin" sounds safe doesn't it. Did you know that according to the centers for disease control (CDC) that aspirin is the 4th deadliest drug in America and the leading cause of kidney disease, and it may thin the blood. Multiple peer reviewed journals say the danger of the aspirin a day far outweigh the perceived benefit. The following is a quote from the Journal of the American Medical Association **"No difference was noted in the incidence of cardiovascular events …irrespective of aspirin use."**

JAMA September 13, 2000;284:1247-1255

Knowing that there are multiple blood thinners other than aspirin that won't harm the kidneys or brain, there might be a healthier choice. The reason aspirin is prescribed so often is because it is a "standard of care" no matter that there may be healthier choices. How about Healthier questions like :"why is the blood thick?" Or here is a big one "Why does my blood need to be thinned?" And did you know water is one of the best blood thinners out there with no negative side effects "if used in moderation". Just kidding, because at multiple gallons a day even water can be harmful. Did you know that the average person needs 50% of their body weight in ounces every day. That means a 150lb person needs 75oz of clean fresh water every day. Tea, coffee and soda don't count. The majority of people I see are not getting close to the healthy amount of water they need. Without the right amount of water you can have a huge number of diagnoses or diseases that can be cured from a good amount of water intake. I encourage you to read "Your bodies many cries for water" by Dr. Batamanghelidj. Brilliant and well researched book on diseases cured by sufficient water intake. A quote from another of Dr. Batamanghelidj books "Water cures drugs kill" he is speaking about the up-coming paradigm shift when the medical world realizes that the symptom= drug approach does more harm than good. "All of a sudden they will feel naked... They see the many years of learning and memorizing "scientific jargons", all the statistical analysis for justification of treatment protocols using toxic chemicals or invasive procedures, and the price structure attached to these acquired skills is declared obsolete." (Dr. Batmanghelidj "Water cures drugs kill")

Armed with the knowledge contained within this book you will be able to make choices that will give you a healthier and more vital life!

Case #2 Debbie a 43 year old mother of 3 children, happily married, diagnosed with High blood pressure at 35 years old, with reflux at 37, with insomnia at 39, with thyroid problems at 40 and fibromyalgia at 42. She was prescribed: 1 drug for high blood pressure, 1 for sleep, 1 for depression (she was told it was for sleep), 1 for indigestion, 1 muscle relaxant, 1 for pain. She was following the doctor's orders and was taking her 6 medications daily, but she still felt bad. When taking her history during her exam she said she had an auto accident when she was 25 years old and she was pregnant at the same time. She felt like she wasn't hurt so she got no care. Her x-ray showed rotation and buckling of her cervical (neck) area. This was causing her nervous system to be in a sympathetic dominant or fight-or-flight state. We started correcting her spinal subluxations (vertebrae out of place causing dangerous pressure on the nerves), changed her diet to eliminate polyunsaturated fatty acids, and eliminate packaged foods. It took 2 weeks for her blood pressure to normalize without the medications, 4 weeks for her reflux to correct, and 3 weeks for her sleep and diffuse joint pain to be nearly eliminated. (NOTE) She made permanent changes in her lifestyle and her family also made those changes, now Debbie is healthy and dynamic and drug free and so is her family. You have to love and honor mom's who take charge!!!

How Your Body Works and Crazy Interventions That Don't Work

Physiology is how the body works. Your body has millions of electrical and chemical processes going on every second. These processes not only keep you alive, without normal physiology you develop Dis-eases. Maintaining normal physiology is Vital. Any food, chemical or activity that changes physiology can make you healthier or sicker. Medications alter physiology, most medications slow or stop metabolic processes and your body is a sea of metabolic processes. This is why, in those crazy drug adds that tell what wonderful benefits this drug or that drug can give you, then rattle off the side effects rapidly. The marketing people don't want you to think critically, they just want you to wander into your doctor and "ask is this drug right for you". This is called Direct To Consumer (DTC) marketing which is illegal in most countries around the world. DTC is great marketing to sell those patentable chemicals called medications but it is NOT health care.

Pharmageddon has been defined as, "the prospect of a world in which medicines and medications produce more ill-health than health, and when medical progress does more harm than good". Ivan Illich warned of the risks of medicalisation, the generally dehumanizing and damaging effects of professional interventions: "*the medical establishment has become a major threat to health*". Mr. Illich was so right when he saw that the medical system was composed of treating symptoms with medications with no regard to the cause of the symptoms, he knew that system was doing more harm than good.

Medications rarely, if ever, address the underlying cause of what is wrong with the person. To treat symptoms with medications without going after the cause of the problem can lead to disaster. If you think about it, medications chemically alter physiology.We have held a belief as a society that medications are based in science and have benefit. That type of "health care" or belief system has lead to the most medicated population the world has ever seen, not the healthiest population just the most drugged. The U.S.A. has 5% of the world's population and consumes 50% of the world's prescriptions. Are Americans just sicker than the rest of the planet or just the most medicated population on earth. Do those medications or chemicals make us healthier and more vital? According to the Journal of the American Medical Association: approximately "106,000 people die each year in U.S. Hospitals from properly prescribed drugs.

Over 2 million suffer serious side effects."(JAMA, 1998).The world health organization rates the health of the population of the U.S.A. 72nd out of 191 countries, 50th in life span and 49th in infant mortality (that is the ability of a child to survive 1 year). Our healthcare is not the best in the world it's far from it. The only category the U.S.A. is #1 is in spending on health care.We spend the most on health care and if we got the best results, I think our population would be happy with the cost. When you look at all of the dialysis centers, the assisted living centers, the epidemic of Alzheimer's, and with 14% of our children in special needs programs, and autism is affecting 1 in 33 boys, its time to rethink what we call "health care". We don't really have a health care system in this country, what we really have is a dis-ease management system. Like Bill Maher stated "…there is no money in healthy people and there is no money in dead people. The money is in the middle, people who are alive, sort of, but with one or more chronic conditions …" A great and terrible wake-up call from the **Partnership to Fight Chronic Disease,**

"The Impact of Chronic Disease on U.S. Health and Prosperity: A Collection of Statistics and Commentary"

- Chronic diseases kill more than 1.7 million Americans per year
- Chronic disease is responsible for 7 of 10 deaths in the U.S.
- 133 million Americans, or 45% of the population, have at least one chronic condition
- 78 million Americans, or 26% have multiple chronic conditions

The above statistics need to scare you into action, our medical system handles symptoms well however the patients don't make out very good. We are just talking about chemically regulating blood pressure and the disasters that that approach cause. It is also true of chemically regulating Cholesterol, or stomach acid, or depression, etc… My whole world when patients come to me is to find the cause. There is a cause of high cholesterol, or a cause of fibromyalgia, or the cause of high blood pressure, which is what this book is about.

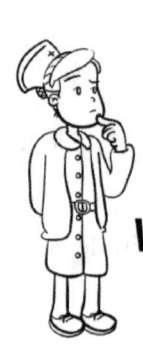 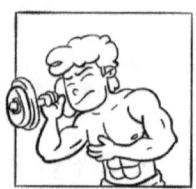 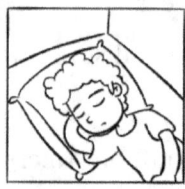

Who has higher blood pressure?

The Body Regulates Itself

What a lot of the doctors forget, and the general public doesn't know, is that blood pressure changes depending on demand and what your body is experiencing at that moment. When more oxygen is needed blood pressure increases, if there is too much carbon dioxide, blood pressure increases, physical, chemical and emotional, stress will also increase blood pressure. Since blood has several functions like bringing oxygen to the tissue and taking away carbon dioxide, or carrying cells vital to your immune system, regulating PH levels, just to name a few of the blood functions. When you slow the flow of blood by decreasing blood pressure chemically, which is the purpose of the drugs that are given if you are diagnosed with high blood pressure. You also decrease the functions of blood. Imaging you decrease oxygen to the tissue or lessen nutrients to the body or you don't remove the waste products fast enough. Would you get decreased energy, dizziness, swelling of legs, increased pain? All are the effects, also called side effects, of blood pressure drugs. Just look at the side effects on the package insert of all medications, and you will see the effects on altering your physiology with that "chemical" or medication. To start to change your perception and regain or maintain vital health, start looking at medications as what they are, they are patentable chemicals designed to alter physiology. Changing your perception is vital to changing your health. For an example if you look at diet coke as cool refreshing and delicious you will keep drinking it. However if you have the knowledge that diet coke has a chemical sweetener that causes neurologic damage and a host of toxic effects on your physiology, you will eliminate that chemical from your diet. The effects of lowering blood pressure with a chemical or medication (if you haven't changed your perception) you have a number of effects like decreasing oxygen to the brain. Could that be one of the reasons we have an epidemic of Alzheimer's today? Knowing that your little 3lb brain burns 25% of your total bodies oxygen. Could over medication of our population be one of the underlying causes of the Alzheimer's epidemic today? By learning, or relearning for health care professionals, how your body regulates blood pressure we may be able to stop this epidemic of over prescription in our U.S.A.. Once you understand the "why" behind your bodies functions you will have a new found appreciation for yourself and how your body works. There is a brilliance with how the body works and a danger by second guessing and over-riding physiology with medications. I have approached my patients with the idea in mind that the body is intelligent. Using this understanding of an innate or inborn intelligence in the body that governs all physiology and just educating patient about the cause of high blood pressure, blood pressure can be brought to a healthy level in a very short time without medications. I want you to come to the realization that you are brilliant, and your body is truly self healing and self regulating. With digestion, elimination, tissue repair, blood pressure regulation, and a host of millions of processes going on without you needing to think about it. You truly are amazing, for an example just think about it, if you cut your finger you don't have to stop and concentrate on repairing the injury. Once skin is broken histamines are released, blood flow to the injury is increased, immune system cells are released, a scab forms and new tissue grows beneath so in a few days all that remains is a small scar. Thousands of cellular processes take place to repair that cut in a beautiful harmony. My intention is for you to develop an appreciation for how wonderful you are and I want you to develop a respect for your physiology. Next time you walk by a mirror look at your reflection and smile, you are made in the image and likeness of God.

Case #3 Bob 56 year old father of 3 children, married for 22 years and 30 lbs over weight. He worked at an office as a manager for 25 years, high stress with little physical activity. He was diagnosed with high cholesterol at 43 years old, High blood pressure at 45, and Erectile Dysfunction at 48, and borderline diabetes at 56. He was prescribed statins for Cholesterol, 2 blood pressure medications, metformin for beginning diabetic, and Viagra for ED. He came to see me for headaches and intermittent low back pain. His exam and x-rays showed grade 2 arthritis which means he has had spinal damage for years. His co-pay for his medications was over $350.00 per month, he actually told me if he got off his meds he would use the extra money to buy a Harley Davidson motorcycle. Care started immediately within 2 weeks his blood pressure began to be normal with reduced medications and his erectile function returned when he reduced his blood pressure medications. It took him 30 days to normalize his blood sugar and blood pressure without medications. His headaches and low back pain was reduced 70% in duration and frequency within 4 weeks and eliminated by 8 weeks of care. He got his motorcycle at 3 months of care. He and his wife are enjoying long motorcycle rides on the coast. He is drug free pain free and happy.

The History of Measuring High Blood Pressure

When talking about blood pressure we should start at the beginning. The history of how blood pressure is taken today began in 1905 when Dr. Nicolai Korotkoff announced a new method to determine blood pressure. Korotkoff found that by using a measured air pressured cuff around an extremity that closed off blood flow and as the cuff deflated he heard different noises--snapping, murmur-like noises, and muffled tones.

Since then there are several different theories for what causes Korotkoff sounds:

the cavitation theory
the arterial wall theory
the turbulence theory
the transmission of heart sounds theory
the water hammer theory

How blood pressure is taken and has been taken for over a hundred years, goes as follows: an air cuff is tightened until blood flow stops then the pressure of the cuff is slowly released and the person taking the blood pressure listens for a sound. When they hear the sound they quickly mark that cuff pressure number down and that is the first number called "systolic". They keep releasing the pressure while listening until the sound they hear stops and then they quickly write that cuff pressure number down and that is the second number called "Diastolic". So the old joke was "to lower your blood pressure get a doctor who is hard of hearing." So Blood pressure is written as systolic / diastolic. It's generally thought that the first number is the output of the heart and the second number is the overall pressure of the body.

The main trouble with checking blood pressure is that your blood pressure increases and decreases constantly. Look at blood pressure as just a snap shot in time or just the pressure at that moment, that is required to stem the flow of blood in your extremity. For example, under straining, a weight lifter can generate 400/200, which is a huge blood pressure number if he was at rest but normal under that strain of lifting. If high blood pressure was always dangerous we would see warning labels on all exercise equipment. "Stay away from that stair stepper, your blood pressure will go up"or "Back away from those bar bells, don't you know lifting those will give you high blood pressure". Have you ever seen a weight lifter straining to lift a bar bell? His face grimaces, he sweats as the weight comes off of the ground. Does he put the weight down and say "I just got a head ache from the blood pressure increase." No, that is just ignorant; High Blood Pressure is NOT a disease. Your body is self-regulating and your body will increase or decrease blood pressure as needed.

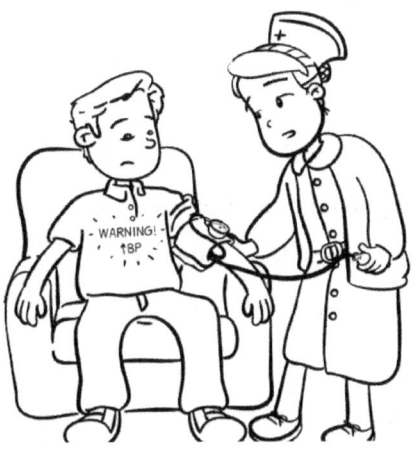

The Real Reason You Need To Measure Blood Pressure

Now here is the real reason we should monitor blood pressure. It is a good indicator of the health of the blood or the health of the arteries. To say "high blood pressure causes strokes" is like saying "cock roaches cause garbage". Cock roaches are attracted to dirty and filthy environments. If every time you saw a dead animal on the side of the road and you saw flies around the dead animal you could say the flies caused the death. Attacking the flies to protect other animals makes about as much logic as lowering blood pressure without understanding what caused it to go up. Most strokes and heart disease come from toxic lifestyles that lead to unhealthy blood and unhealthy arteries so blood pressure will change depending on what is going on with the body. We are going to go over what dangerous circumstance causes blood pressure to go up. Because if you know what causes high blood pressure you can go after the source of why your body has raised it and you will be able to change the cause and have a longer healthier more vital life.

What needs to be understood is that the body is self healing and self regulating. That means the body regulates itself! I know I keep repeating this phrase "self-regulating" but this information, and you owning this, will mean the difference between life and death. Yep That means Blood pressure just like every other function from how your body repairs a broken bone or torn skin or how you digest that delicious vegetable shepherd's pie you had last night for dinner. You will break down your dinner to regenerate and rebuild your body. You will break down the proteins to amino acids, the fats to fatty acids and the carbohydrates to usable sugars. All of these functions are done automatically by the autonomic nervous system controlling the amazing systems that are your body.

The Beauty of Your Automatic Nervous System

This autonomic nervous system is what helps regulate blood
pressure. A brief overview of this system is it's composed of
two parts, one keeps you alive under stress called "the fight
or flight system" also called the sympathetic nervous system.
The other part is called "the rest digest and repair system"
also the parasympathetic system. When one system is
activated the other is essentially deactivated. Imagine that
you were resting in an easy chair and all of a sudden an
unexpected loud bang goes off, someone cuts you off in
traffic, working out at the gym, or any stressful circumstance
your fight or flight system is activated. So stress activates this
fight or flight system. You can boil all stressors down to
physical, chemical, or emotional causes. What is wild is, your
body doesn't know the difference between physical, chemical
or emotional stressors it kicks in this fight or flight system to
keep you alive in the short term. To protect you in the short
term this system raises your heart rate, reduces blood supply
to the gut or digestion, decreases your immune system and
increases LDL Cholesterol (this type of Cholesterol is called
"bad Cholesterol" by some doctors who forget it has a major
functions like it's used for tissue repair and is the precursor to

stress hormones). So when this fight or flight system is on people may be misdiagnosed with high blood pressure, high blood sugar, high cholesterol, digestive problems, etc… I say misdiagnosed because the underlying cause of the problem was not identified.

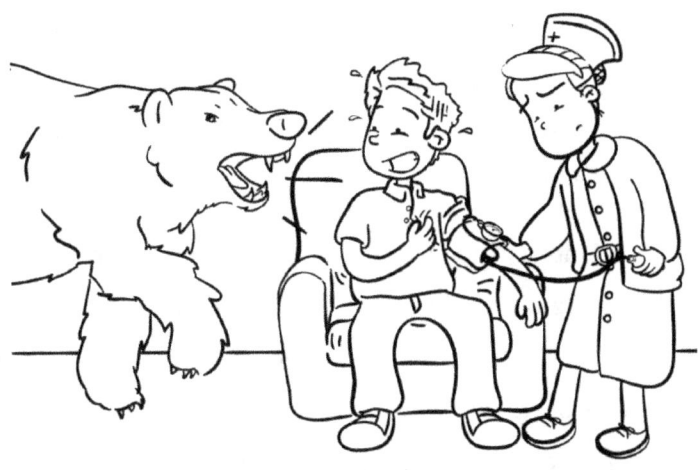

Stress the Real Cause of High Blood Pressure

This is vital that you really understand that blood pressure will increase or decrease in response to stressors or the lack of stressors. The underlying cause of physical, chemical or emotional stress is almost always missed in today's medical system. Physical stress could be chronic pain or a sedentary life style. Chemical stress could be poor diet, dehydration, over medication (the average American over 60 years old is on 12 prescriptions). Emotional stress is based on your perception of situations. Let's say you love roller coasters (I'm scared of them) so if you went on a thrill ride you would get off of it elated I would get off of that ride with abject terror. Your immune system would be stimulated, my immune system would be depressed. We went thru the same experience just a different perception and a totally different physical response.

 So much emphasis today is on having "low blood pressure" and this thought that blood pressure should be low is reinforced by the majority of the medical community and the media. This pervasive view that low blood pressure is healthy is making a sick overly medicated population. If a doctor prescribes you a drug to lower your blood pressure ask "why is my blood pressure high" or "what is broken with my body's blood pressure regulating system" or here is a big question that will save your life "will this drug make me live longer and healthier". Now that last one was just plain mean because the answer will usually be a lie. You see people typically with low blood pressure do live longer in most circumstances. Even though in some health conditions a higher blood pressure will give you a longer life. Like this study from the Journal of the American Medical Association:

 "Mortality rates were more than four times higher for those with systolic pressures of less than 120, in comparison to those who had pressure over 161 systolic.

These conclusions were gleaned from research on more than 48,000 heart failure patients seen at 259 U.S. hospitals between March 2003 and December 2004.

Journal of the American Medical Association November 8, 2006; 296(18): 2217-2226

This study involving more than 48,000 heart failure patients on the surface sounds crazy. Unless you know the body is self-regulating and self-healing. Why would the body increase blood pressure in people who have had heart damage? Let's look at this logically. If your heart was damaged, like in heart failure, do you think that maybe the arteries may not be healthy. I know that is me stating the obvious. So to keep the same amount of oxygen and nutrients through damaged tissue your body may have to increase the pressure to keep your tissue and body alive. So after this study, did all of the medical doctors change their dogmatic views and start to look at why their patients have high blood pressure. Nope our medical system is like a giant ship going full speed and for this baby to change direction or change policy, it takes a lot of time to pass or a lot of lives have to be lost. Just look at the pain reliever Vioxx® this drug was passed out for years and it killed more people than died in the Vietnam war before it was taken off of the market. There was no one indicted in those medication caused deaths, at most it was just a slight mention on the evening news. The public didn't storm the pharmaceutical companies with pitch forks. The Vioxx® scandal was just one example of deaths caused by properly prescribed medications. There are hundreds of other examples, the medical world is full of medications and procedures that have been hailed, when they were first started, as the best, the newest, the most advanced. Only to be taken off of the market after it was found out that the damage caused by the drug or procedure was greater than any perceived benefit. To alter physiology with a chemical (medication) can be disastrous especially when the patient is taking multiple medications with unknown reactions when they are taken together. For an example: If a pain reliever is taken for say joint pain do you really think that drug goes to a joint and fixes a problem? That drug, just like all medications, goes thru your digestive system, filtered by your liver then carried by your blood stream throughout your body affecting every system. To know the truth of what effects a medication can cause in your body just look at the "side effects" written in micro print on the package inserts. If you are getting your information about a drug from television you have to listen fast because the effects are said really, really fast half way through the drug commercials. Those commercials are comedic if you look beyond the glitz. Picture a young healthy person running thru a beautiful field after taking the allergy medication and the announcer says "this may cause kidney disease, weakening of your immune system, etc... " Then you always get the "Ask your doctor if this is right for you". That is just nuts, how about we change that system and respect the body and its physiology. We are only going to explore blood pressure regulation with this book however please apply what you learn here to every medication or diagnosis you have been given.

Case #4 Lori: a 68 year old woman mother of 2 children, grandmother of 4 children. Diagnosed with scoliosis as a teenager (she received no care at that time for her scoliosis). She had chronic pain her whole life so she was given NSAIDs like Advil®, Motrin®, etc. After taking the pain medications for years she developed gastrointestinal problems. Over the next several years she was diagnosed with high blood pressure, depression, severe reflux, sleep problems, and chronic pain. She was taking 9 prescriptions when she came into my clinic. After her exam and x-rays I was excited to find that her 37degree scoliosis could be reduced. Care started immediately. Within 30 days her blood pressure was normal without medications, within 2 weeks her pain was reduced to a manageable level and within 6 months of care her 37 degree scoliosis was reduced to 27 degrees. She was able to eliminate all of her medications over the next year. She is now able to play golf, walk daily, and she said "she got her life back". Just imagine the courage she took to break free of the medical system she had been in for over 50years. Lori You ROCK!!!

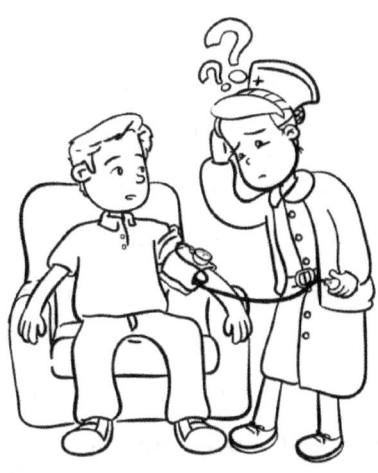

The Importance of the "Why" Behind Your Symptoms

The current medical system is not concerned with the "why" behind changes in physiology or blood pressure. The current view is that everyone should have one blood pressure. I know it sounds stupid that an 18 year old athlete should have the same blood pressure as the 60 year old overweight person. Especially considering that for every one pound of extra fat there is one mile of blood vessels. That means a person 20lbs over weight has 20 miles more to pump blood through. To keep the same amount of oxygen flowing to an overweight person do you think the heart should increase pressure? To medicate that overweight person to a lower blood pressure does that make that person healthier? Will they live longer? Will they have more energy and a better quality of life? These questions need to be asked and answered for optimal vital health to be achieved. The idea that everyone should have a blood pressure within a narrow range is illogical and unscientific and has lead us to the most drugged culture the world has ever seen. I like the old medical text book quote **"The first principle of the therapy of hypertension is the knowledge of when to treat and when not to treat."**.. Harrison's Medical Text book.

We used to have a view that the top number (systolic) should be 100 plus your age. That was the standard medical view for decades. It was understood that generally as you age your arteries get less flexible so systolic pressure has to increase. To say nothing about if your diet or lifestyle is toxic the arteries could be damaged and your body may have to increase pressure to keep the same amount of oxygen and nutrients flowing to keep you healthy. So the "why" behind any high blood pressure diagnosis is a question that, quite literally, your life depends on. Our current medical system rarely asks. The "why" behind disease.

The paradigm shift of "Why"

Like why does a person suddenly develop "high blood pressure" or "high cholesterol"? Could the high blood pressure just be the body adapting to arteries that are damaged or blood that is toxic? Is high cholesterol a disease or, since cholesterol has several functions such as immune system or tissue repair, could high cholesterol levels be a sign that there is stress or tissue damage? To lower either blood pressure or cholesterol without knowing the cause you will experience a loss of health and a weakening of your natural body's responses to fighting disease. What we end up with is not health care but disease management. The new life-saving paradigm shift that is taking place is people are asking "Why". People are beginning to question their doctors and the therapies the doctors are recommending.

Peter sterling from Cambridge said it best in his paper titled "**Principles of Allostasis: optimal design, predictive regulation, pathophysiology and rational therapeutics.**" *Yep that is the title.* Here is a quote from this brilliant paper "In medicine, major diseases now rise in prevalence, such as essential hypertension and type 2 diabetes, whose causes the homeostasis model cannot explain....**And treating these diseases with drugs to fix low-level mechanisms that are not broken turns out not to work particularly well."** The highlights are mine, in typical British under statement. According to (Dangerous Drugs, 1992). "In an average year, 1.6 million people are hospitalized due to the side effects of prescribed drugs. Up to 160,000 will die from their reaction".

So does that mean that even high blood pressure may mean that the body is adapting to a health challenge such as toxic unhealthy blood or damaged arteries? Absolutely. Doctors today are caught between "a rock and a hard place". Our medical system is based on fear. We have a system that Doctors have their hands tied in many circumstances because of "treatment protocols". For example let's say that a patient is prescribed an Aspirin a day, for a "healthy heart" ..Riiight. Now aspirin is the 4th deadliest drug in America and the leading cause of kidney disease. According to the New England Journal of Medicine December 20, 2001

"Individuals who have kidney disease or other ailments who regularly take aspirin or acetaminophen (main ingredient in

Tylenol ®) may be boosting their risk of developing kidney failure. ....The results support those of other studies that have found an association between regular use of painkillers and an increased risk of chronic kidney failure in susceptible individuals." Another name for kidney failure is Death! Are there better more effective ways of dealing with symptoms like pain or high blood pressure without risking death?

We have to go back to respecting the intelligent nature of the body. The most common pain relievers prescribed for joint pain are a class of drugs called Non-Steroidal Anti-inflammatories or NSAIDs. However one of the effects is that they destroy the building blocks of cartilage. According to the American Journal of Medicine, 1999, Dec, NSAIDs:

✖ Decrease cartilage production

✖ Inhibits proteoglycan production (the building blocks of cartilage)

✖ Causes accelerated bone destruction

So for a recap: NSAIDs cause bone destruction and stop the building blocks of cartilage and it is given to people with joint pain. Is that ethical, moral, or even scientific? Today that ignorant drugging of symptoms is passed off as quality medical care. Those are just some pain relievers and some of the effects, just like how blood pressure drugs don't address the cause, pain relievers never address the source of why the body is giving you pain. I have had thousands of patients with every type of pain you could imagine , headaches, neuropathy (nerve problems), Neuralgia (nerve pain), sciatica, foot pain, carpal tunnel syndrome, etc…None of those patients had a medication deficiency. All of the patients had an underlying cause and when that cause was addressed the symptoms resolved. Here is something you need to burn into your soul; Your Body Raises Blood Pressure in Response to Pain!!!

There are many books on disease reversal thru nutrition and/or detoxing. Such as " There is a cure for Diabetes" By Dr Gabriel Cousins, "Reversing Heart Disease" By Dr Julian Whittaker, "Prostate Health in 90 days" by Dr Larry Clapp.

The list is endless of the Doctors who have found effective solutions for reversing disease. So if there are cures out there how come your family doctor doesn't know about them? And why isn't this practiced by your regular doctor? The answer is in your doctors training. There is very little emphasis in medical school on the wisdom of the human body and the ability of it to reverse disease. There is a huge push for the dogma of the germ theory and pharmaceutical therapies AKA drugs. Most people don't know the details about the "germ theory". I like this quote from Etienne de Harven M.D. about Virus mania:

"Virus Mania is a social disease of our highly developed society. To cure it will require conquering fear, fear being the most deadly contagious virus, most efficiently transmitted by the media. *Errare humanum est sed diabolicum preservare…* (to err is human, but to preserve an error is diabolic)."

The Germ concept is that germs cause disease, now it is true that germs are present in diseased tissue it is also true that germs are present in healthy tissue. A contemporary of Pasteur, Professor Estor, remarked "Bacteria cannot be the cause of gangrene; they are the effects of it." For an infection to occur there has to be a weakening of the immune system. The main reason the medical world keeps trying to fight germs is the alternative is to strengthen the immune system. Which medications can't do. Prescription medications don't strengthen the immune system, only healthy food, vitamins and minerals strengthen the immune system and the standard medical doctor of today has little to no training in nutrition.

So the medical system continues to fight germs instead of strengthen the immune system.

Now I would be behind Drug therapy if the cause of the suffering was lack of drugs!! Heck I would be promoting drugs if that was an effective method for health. The real research doesn't back up that approach. When I get a patient in who is taking multiple prescriptions I tell them to separate the drugs and to never take 2 drugs together and try to separate them by at least an hour and drink a whole glass of water between to lessen the negative effects. The response I usually get is "Doc there aren't enough hours in the day to do that" Then I will tell them "to take one of every drug they were prescribed grind them up together and take that concoction to the police and ask if the person that gave them that was trying to kill them or if it's safe". Universally Patients laugh and say "of course they will say its poison". I even had a patient say "police don't prescribe so they wouldn't know, that is why his doctor is keeping track of his medications". Some people have such a blind faith in the wisdom of the medical doctor and the protocols they follow that even though they get sicker and sicker year after year from taking medications they just keep following the orders. This book is dedicated to those patients that are breaking from this "Matrix", just like that movie, once you learn the truth you can never go back to the old reality. Once you realize that you are self-regulating and self-healing then you will look at what you put in your body is important. Many cultures pray before meals for 2 reasons to give thanks for the food and second to honor what you are eating will truly become you. That is a wild concept, think of it would you rather be made of a diet coke and chicken nugget or spring water and sweet honeydew melon. It is your choice!

You see I need that type of a pattern interrupt to get my patients and people I meet to realize the insanity and lack of science behind what they think is "Health Care" when in reality it is at best "disease management" and has nothing to do with correcting that cause of the symptoms. Health isn't lack of symptoms.

If I drop a brick on my foot it should hurt. That is a symptom letting me know that I have damaged tissue. If my blood was toxic or my nerves were compressed I could drop that brick on my foot and not feel it. That's why some people who have toxic blood that destroy the nerves ability to transmit info to the brain called diabetes have lost the feeling in their feet. This is called "neuropathy" a combination or Latin words "neuro" or nerve and "pathy" or problem in English it would be a nerve problem.

A lot of doctors use Latin terms to describe symptoms. I once had a patient who had foot pain from weak muscles of his feet and he wanted another opinion so he went to his regular Doc who diagnosed him with "metatarsalgia" which is "metatarsals" (the bones of the foot) and "algia" ('pain' in Latin) so His regular Doctor just gave a diagnosis of Foot pain in Latin.

He was prescribed a pain reliever and he still had the weak muscles but he was more comfortable. When you know that the pain reliever that he was prescribed was a non-steroidal anti-inflammatory or NSAIDs and those inhibits prostaglandin formation clumping blood cells together and leading to a destruction of cartilage or degeneration of his joints. Gee doesn't that sound like good medical care???

Here is a study from the Archives of Internal Medicine that followed more than 80,000 women between the ages of 31 and 50 years who were initially hypertension-free.

- two years later

- women who used NSAIDs 22 days or more per month, the risk of high-blood pressure increased some 86 percent.

"Nonetheless, it was concluded that a large portion of U.S. hypertension cases may be the result of over-using these pain medications"

Archives of Internal Medicine. October 28, 2002;162:2204-2208

The Natural Solution to High Blood Pressure

By now you have the idea that using drugs to lower blood pressure is NOT a good solution so here are the keys that you will need to take blood pressure correctly. **First take it correctly**. Realize that Blood pressure increases or decreases depending on need. Things that raise Blood Pressure are: a cold room, a full bladder, emotional stress (white coat syndrome), not breathing correctly, talking while taking the blood pressure, etc… there are thousands of reasons blood pressure will go up. To drive the point home with my patients I ask them "if they want to take blood pressure while they are riding a bike uphill? Of course they say "No" that it would be high, then I will say, do they want to take the blood pressure while they are weight lifting? Again they will say "No". I have to walk people through these scenario's to plant the seed that blood pressure will go up under natural circumstances.

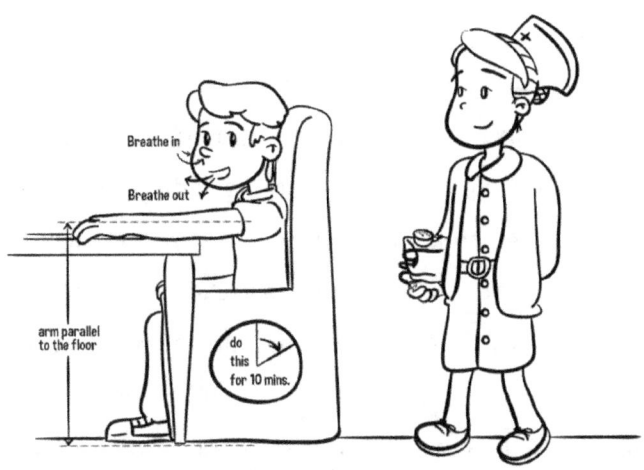

The Anatomy of blood pressure

You have sensors in your neck at the junction where your carotid artery splits into the internal and external carotid arteries. These sensors check carbon dioxide levels and blood pressure levels called the carotid sinus and carotid body. If carbon dioxide levels are high, the blood pressure will be increased to get more blood to your lungs to get rid of the acid called carbon dioxide. You also realize by now that you need to change your physiology to naturally lower your blood pressure and that takes about 10 minutes.

You need to sit with your feet on the floor and breathe deep for 10 minutes. And you have to breathe correctly. When you breathe in your diaphragm contracts and your tummy or abdomen should push out. When you breathe out your diaphragm relaxes and your tummy should move in. This is called by many names "belly breathing" "diaphragmatic breathing" "yoga breathing" it is how we first learned to breathe. You have to relearn how to breathe. Put one hand on your chest (this should not move in relaxed breathing. And place one hand on your tummy (this should move out on inhalation and in on exhalation). This will take practice. You need to sit for 10 minutes and deep breathe correctly with your arm level with your heart, then after 10 minutes check your blood pressure. There is a very cool machine called "RESPeRATE®" that is FDA approved to lower blood pressure "when medications are not effective". All it does is cause you to deep breathe for 15 minutes. And this according to the advertisement "will lower blood pressure all day long". I would recommend you save the $300 cost of RESPeRATE® and just learn to breathe correctly. Yep that's right you need 10 minutes to take blood pressure correctly.

The Nutrition Behind Good Blood Pressure

In the U.S.A. today we have a population that is obese and starving at the same time. This is a population that's starving for healthy nutrients. Any time you see somebody with an excess of a human body or obese, what they're doing is taking in nutrients that they're not digesting. So the body is storing it. Since the standard American diet is loaded with toxic fats, Genetically Modified Organisms (GMO's), preservatives, and chemical flavorings, this means that the population is toxic. So, we have to deal with the toxicities in correcting high blood pressure. We have to eliminate GMO's. There are no human studies but there are a few animal studies that show:

Identified health risks associated with GM food consumption, including:

- ✖ Infertility
- ✖ Immune system compromise
- ✖ Accelerated aging

Altered genes associated with:

- ✖ cholesterol synthesis,
- ✖ insulin regulation,
- ✖ cell signaling,
- ✖ protein formation

Alterations in:

✖ liver, kidney, spleen and gut function

Many countries in the world are not allowing GMO crops in because of the known health risks and the unknown consequences to human consumption. However in U.S.A. The approved GMs in the U.S. include:

Herbicide resistance

✖ Corn, soy, cotton, canola, rice, alfalfa, beet, flax

Insect resistance (Pesticide prod)

✖ Corn, cotton, potato, tomato

Sterile pollen (Terminator Tech)

✖ Corn, chicory

Virus resistance

✖ Papaya, squash, plum

Delayed ripening

✖ Tomato

Altered oil

✖ Canola, soy

Protein composition

✖ Corn

Reduced nicotine tobacco

The only way to be safe and not to consume toxic food is to get 100% organic food. That is another essential requirement for recovery from high blood pressure.

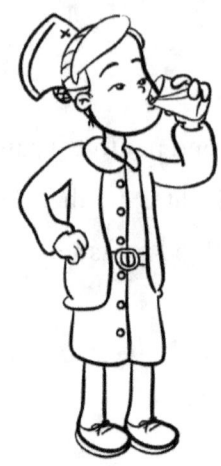

Clear Clean Water

To start with, you need to be fully hydrated that means you need healthy water about 50% of your body weight in ounces every day. That means a 200 lb person needs 100 ounces of water every day. Remember water is a good blood thinner. The main problem with the water most people are exposed to is toxins. Water today is fluoridated, chlorinated, or packaged in toxic containers. Filtering today's water is vital to your survival. Water packaged in plastic containers is not regulated by the FDA unless it crosses state lines. I encourage everyone to watch the movie "Tapped" on what is happening with the bottled water industry. You need to first filter out the fluoride and use a filter that eliminates chloride, chlorine, heavy metals, bacteria, and drugs too. Healthy water is the key to healthy metabolic function and below is a talk I gave on the importance of healthy water.

https://www.youtube.com/watch?v=nb6ttXxb5tU

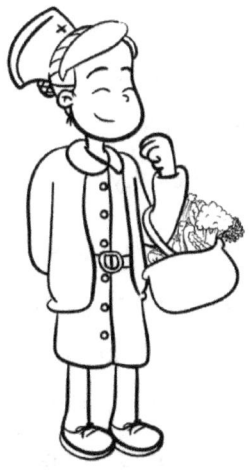

Plant and Unprocessed Diet Vital for Health

Your diet needs to be 80% plant based minimum, and organic. The reason plant based is important is because there are endotoxins on animal products that can cause systemic inflammation. This will thicken the blood and increase blood pressure. A plant based diet also has fibers that clean the arteries.

Eliminate the Poly Unsaturated Fatty Acids also called PUFAs. PUFAs are in almost all packaged foods, they include canola oil, soy oil, safflower oil, and most seed oils. PUFAs cause blood cells to clump together. Blood cells are shaped like a biconcave disc, like 2 Frisbees® glued together.

This design holds the maximum amount of oxygen. If the blood cells are clumped together they can't hold a good amount of oxygen and the blood gets thicker so pressure has to increase to get that unhealthy blood through the arteries.

For normal physiology you need to get lots of fresh organic fruits and vegetables, and eliminate gluten and eliminate dairy. This is the solution to healthy self-regulation and self-healing. Eliminate any genetically modified foods, in fact if man makes it, don't eat it. Since it takes about 90 days to heal a gut for 90 days eliminate packaged or canned foods, no fast foods, and no animal products (meats and dairy).Try and get your food as organic and fresh as possible. The gut is typically very damaged in patients with high blood pressure so you may have to predigest your food to ease off pressure on the digestive system. By predigesting I mean, juicing and blending. This process breaks down the plants better than chewing and makes it easier to get the healing nutrients out of your food. For healthy nutrition and to clean your arteries you need both a blender and a juicer. The best blender is a Blendtec® or a Vitamix® I have the Blendtec® and I love it. For the best juicer I have tried the Champion juicer®, Breville juicer®, Green Star juicer®, and the Omega VRT-350 juicer®. My Favorite is the Omega VRT-350 juicer®.

The difference between juicing and blending is that a juicer separates the heavy fibers or insoluble fibers from the small fibers or the soluble fibers. A blender uses the whole plant and most blenders are typically high speed. The advantages of a blender are you use the whole plant so this is great for smoothies. And blenders are great for fruits, because with most fruits you want to use the whole fruit to get the best benefits. The disadvantage of blenders is that the high speed tends to oxidize the juice and may destroy some enzymes and it doesn't separate the insoluble fibers from the soluble fibers. This process of getting the soluble fibers separated is vital for cleaning arteries. Heavy fibers are great for cleaning the intestinal track and very necessary for health. A good formula for juicing I recommend is:

Tasty and nutritious juice formula and this produces about 20, 16oz mason jars of juice:

3 X 3lb bags of Apples,

2 X 5 lb bags of carrots

6 bundles of Spinach

3 bundles of celery

Put the juice in mason jars and over fill them so when you

put the tops on there are no air pockets and refrigerate them right away. They should stay fresh for between 24 to 72 hours depending on the juicer. High speed juicer will introduce a lot of oxygen and degrade the juice faster where a slow speed masticating juicer will make the juice stay fresher longer. Get creative on juicing, use a variety. When you are preparing broccoli save the stalks for juice, in fact most of the veggie parts that you would normally throw away may be good for your juice. The reason I like the formula above is apples have malic acid which is great for cleaning arteries and leave the core in the apple when you juice. The spinach is loaded with protein, the carrots help with lung function for detoxing, and celery is great for minerals. Add anything you want: Kale, fennel, any dark green veggies.

Blending is great for fruits , you need to blend not juice fruits, apples are an exception you can both blend and juice apples. Blending is awesome for a fast breakfast or a quick meal. My favorite blending formulas are:

Coconut Smoothie workout / breakfast:

1 young Thai coconut, 1 frozen banana, 1 scoop veggie raw protein powder, 2 tbs raw cacao chips or powder, 1 scoop spiralina.

Here is a video on juicing and blending

http://www.youtube.com/watch?v=INrXthOFQtU

Good oils to use are organic cold pressed olive oil, organic raw coconut oil, or organic palm oil. Healthy fats are vital for healthy thyroid and adrenal function both are needed for healthy blood pressure control. I recommend, on average, about 3 tbs. of coconut oil per day for the average person, follow your doctor's recommendation for oils. Some people may have medical conditions that will cause a difficulty to digest them. Keep in mind though that most doctors have no training in nutrition so make sure your doctor has experience and is educated on the effects of diet and its effect on the disease process. Coconut oil doesn't require a gall bladder for absorption like most other oils so if you have had your gall bladder removed this may be a good option for you. Coconut oil is a medium chain fatty acid it is excellent for healing brain function. A healthy brain burns glucose and if there is a leaky gut present such as most people today who have had antibiotics, vaccinations, or exposure to pesticides in commercially produced foods the coconut oil acts as a second source of brain energy. If you have leaky gut syndrome the large proteins usually gluten (from grains) and caseins (from dairy) can attach to opiate receptors (pleasure sensors) in the brain. This action of blocking the receptor sites is very common in patients with high blood pressure and Attention Deficit Disorder (ADD), and common in Autism Spectrum Disorders (ASD) and FMS. This causes an almost starving of the brain. So it is essential to go on a gluten free / dairy free diet and get at least 1tbs. to 5tbs of raw organic coconut oil a day to heal the brain.

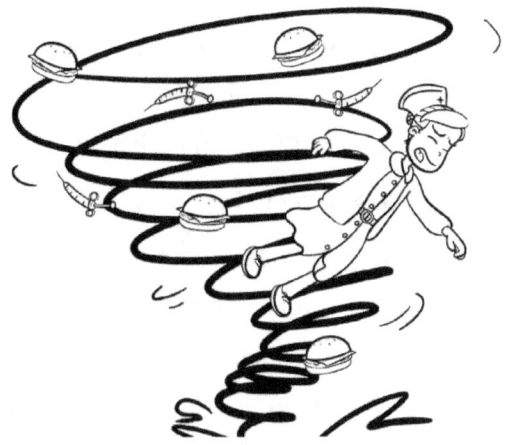

The Perfect Storm of Toxic Vaccinations and Neurotoxins

Case #5 "The perfect storm" : Todd an 11 year old boy diagnosed with headaches for 5 years and high blood pressure for 1 year. He had a common birth in this country (not normal). His mom was given a flu shot when she was pregnant. Now there have been no studies to show that it is safe for a pregnant women to get a flu shot. There are even a number of research papers calling this medical procedure unsafe for children, it still goes on. Todd was born in a hospital and his mom was given an injection of Pitocin to stimulate contractions. Now this injection interrupts the natural birth rhythm between the mother and child. So

Todd's head was jammed against the cervix during the strong uterine contractions caused by the Pitocin. Then when he was born he was injected with the hepatitis B vaccine, even though he was not at risk of hepatitis B. This is not done in most countries of the world but is part of our welcome to America. With the trauma to his neck during the birth process Todd developed ear infections. Now even though the recommendation from the American Board of Pediatrics is to not give antibiotics right away for ear pain and mild swelling of the ear drum he was given 3 rounds of antibiotics during his childhood. This caused damage to his gastrointestinal tract causing leaky gut. Now his mother was recommended by her obstetrician to give him a soy based formula. Now think of this this is a genetically modified soy (never been tested on humans) mixed with fluoridated water (damaging to the brain and thyroid) the microwaved in plastic (with known carcinogens leaching into the baby food) then he got the full recommended vaccination schedule of:

81vaccines by the time he was six years old.

- ✖ **Birth**: Hepatitis B   **1**
  Vaccine
- ✖ **2 Months**: DPT, Polio, Hib, Hep B   **6 Vaccines**
- ✖ **4 Months**: DPT, Polio, Hib   **5 Vaccines**

- ✖ **6 Months**: DPT, Hib   **4 Vaccines**
- ✖ **6-18 Months**: Hep B   **1 Vaccine**
- ✖ **15-18 Months**: DPT, Polio, Hib, MMR **8 Vaccines**
- ✖ **4-6 Years**: DPT, Polio, MMR   **7 Vaccines**
- ✖ By the time a child is **6 months** old they are to be injected with at least **47** vaccines; at **18** months at least **67**, and at **4-6 years** at least **81!-** *based on the 2009 CDC recommended schedule*

I encourage everyone to do the research themselves. Two of the most well researched doctors are Dr Tim O'Shea http://www.thedoctorwithin.com/ , and Dr Sherri Tenpenny http://drtenpenny.com/ . These courageous doctors are looking at the science breaking from the dogmatic view of most of the medical world. Just like Galileo had an idea that the world revolved around the sun which was totally different than the powers that were in control, he was nearly burned at the stake for speaking the truth. Vaccines are a medical procedure. You should have the right to choose any medical procedure or to decline any medical procedure. I encourage everyone to get educated on this controversial subject I will cover vaccines in future books but now just know that vaccines can contribute to aggravation of symptoms through leaky gut, systemic inflammation, neurotoxicity and molecular mimicry.

Now add this to the vaccine assault, the poisoning by genetically modified foods and the neurotoxins found in commercially produced foods and you have the "perfect storm" of a toxic entrance to life. Now he was diagnosed with high blood pressure. My first question when he came to me was "is he uncomfortable at the medical doctors office" his parents told me he was panicked. This is called "white coat hypertension" When I took his blood pressure it was dangerously low. So I recommended his parents take his blood pressure at home I showed them how to take it correctly and within 3 weeks the doctor that put him on those drugs took him off. We also got him on a healthy diet and corrected subluxation of his upper neck that was casing the ear infections and occasional headaches. He is fine health drug free and a great soccer player.

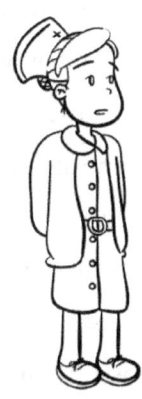 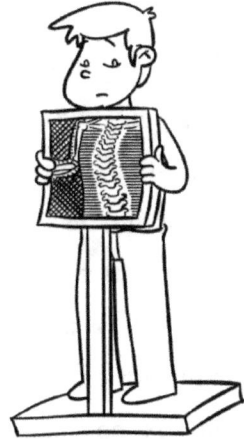

The Physical Stress Behind High Blood Pressure

I have seen hundreds of patients diagnosed with high blood pressure and so far 100% have had some type of cervical (neck) or thoracic (rib cage) stress that is contributing to their high blood pressure. This stress can only be seen on an x-ray and can only be corrected by a Chiropractor who is skilled in correcting subluxations. A subluxation is a vertebra (bones of the spine) that is slightly malpositioned in relation to the vertebra above and below that is affecting the nervous system. Subluxations can have a mechanical effect of decreasing rib motion (vital to breathing) and subluxations can have a neurologic component. Dr. Rodger Speery Nobel

Prize winner said, that posture affects the nervous system. **"90% of your brain's daily activity is involved with positioning your body against gravity"** What that means is that if the posture is altered, that's going to alter sensation, or sensory input into the brain, and the brain controls every function including blood pressure. The medical approach for physical stress is usually: muscle relaxants, pain relievers, anti-inflammatories. And these drugs will mask symptoms but will not fix the underlying cause of a possible subluxation or spinal misalignment. Subluxations are missed because the medical world is NOT trained to reposition the abnormally positioned vertebrae or vertebral subluxation. If they are not trained to fix subluxations they will not look for them or the symptoms caused by that nerve pressure. Abnormal position of a vertebrae causes abnormal motion, abnormal motion causes abnormal proprioceptive signals to the brain. The information sent to the brain will cause the brain to go to the fight or flight state or the rest, digest, and repair mode. Abnormal position of the vertebrae can keep the body in a chronic fight or flight state. This is the most commonly missed finding in high blood pressure, so far, of the hundreds of patients I have seen with high blood pressure, 100% have some evidence of physical trauma causing at least some, if not most, of their symptoms. So correcting the physical source of the symptoms, the patient recovers and gets back to a normal healthy state. If a subluxation is affecting the person, it can cause the sympathetic nervous system or the fight or flight system to be activated. This would increase heart rate, and decrease blood supply to the gut, both will lead the body to have high blood pressure.

Health of Your Blood Vessels Will Effect Blood Pressure

Healthy arteries are flexible and have a spring-ability to them. When the heart contracts, blood pressure has a spike or naturally goes up just like a good pump should. The body uses the natural spring-ability of the arteries to help pump the blood throughout the body. As we age our arteries lose some of their springiness so systolic usually goes up naturally, this is why systolic used to be (and still is in some countries) 100 plus your age. Other factors that cause your arteries to lose their springiness are poor diets. If your arteries are damaged by toxic foods or chemicals the body will protect the arteries with a plaque. Ignorant doctors will call this a disease named atherosclerosis, in reality it is a protective action by the body to tissue damage. To correct this problem you have to clean the arteries. There are basically two types of fiber found in food insoluble and soluble, one will clean the colon the other cleans the arteries. I have seen arteries so badly damaged that you can even see the plaquing on an x-ray. People who have that much damage must get massive amounts of soluble fibers daily to clean the arteries. And you must avoid any foods or additives that can damage the arteries such as MSG. Our food supply is flooded with neurotoxins so for health of your nervous system (which regulates your blood pressure) you have to eliminate those toxins. The most common is an excitotoxin called monosodium glutamate or MSG. MSG is an excitotoxin, which means it overexcites your cells to the point of damage or death, causing brain damage to varying degrees -- and triggering or worsening learning disabilities, ADD, Depression, Bipolar disorders, Alzheimer's disease, Parkinson's disease, Lou Gehrig's disease and more.

MSG is found in many food additives-for example:

Hydrolyzed Protein

Glutamic Acid

Monopotassium Glutamate

Monosodium Glutamate

Textured Protein

Yeast Extract

Autolyzed Yeast

Yeast Food

Yeast Nutrient

Calcium Caseinate

Gelatin

Anything Protein Fortified

Barley Malt

Natural Beef Flavoring

Protease

Corn Starch

Flavors and Flavorings

Seasonings

Natural Flavors and Flavorings

Natural Pork Flavoring

Natural Chicken Flavoring

Soy Sauce

Soy Protein Isolate

Soy Protein

Bouillon

Stock

Broth

Citric Acid

Powdered Milk

Anything Protein Fortified

Anything Enzyme Modified

Malt Extract

Malt Flavoring

Barley Malt

Whey Protein

Carrageenan

Maltodextrin

Pectin

Enzymes

The FDA has allowed this poison into our food supply under multiple different names. For safety I recommend "if man makes it, don't eat it" to my patients. The reason MSG is used because it attaches to the pleasure centers in the brain so anything you mix with this chemical, the brain will perceive as a good flavor. Bad cheap food with a long shelf life will still taste good. MSG is great for the food industry but bad for people. FDA seems to be working for industry and not the safety of health of our population.

A great book on MSG by Dr. Russell Blaylock, a board-certified neurosurgeon and author of *"Excitotoxins: The Taste that Kills."* This is a great read with amazing information.

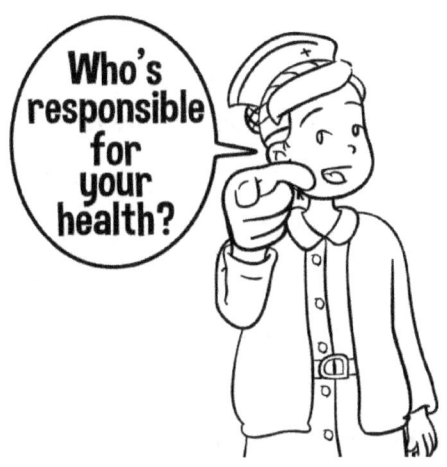

Final Word and Challenge

Like Albert Einstein said, "We cannot solve our problems with the same thinking we used when we created them." It may be hard to deal with the health care "professionals" that gave you the medications that alter your natural physiology. They are educated in a system that is broken. It takes a tremendous amount of courage and action to break the drug slavery that most Americans are enduring. Do NOT stop your medications on your own, that can be deadly. Find a Doctor who understands physiology and goes after the causes of why your body is presenting with symptoms. I hold this belief that you are made in the image and likeness of God, you are self-regulating and self-healing. You should smile every time you walk by a mirror. I am blessed a thousand times over for my connection with my patients and all my friends that I have met through the internet. This is a worldwide movement to appreciate your light and that unseen life force within. You have an innate, inborn intelligence that can reverse disease and give you the greatest full dynamic life ever. You just have to know the basics in anatomy, physiology, nutrition, and the toxins to avoid. My hope is that the information in this book will help you on the path to achieve optimal health and a full life of at least 120 years.

God Bless

Dr. John Bergman D.C.

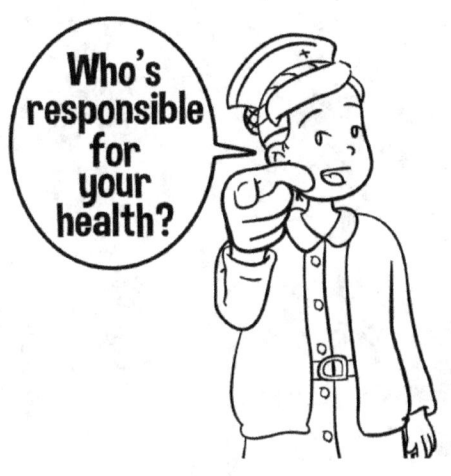

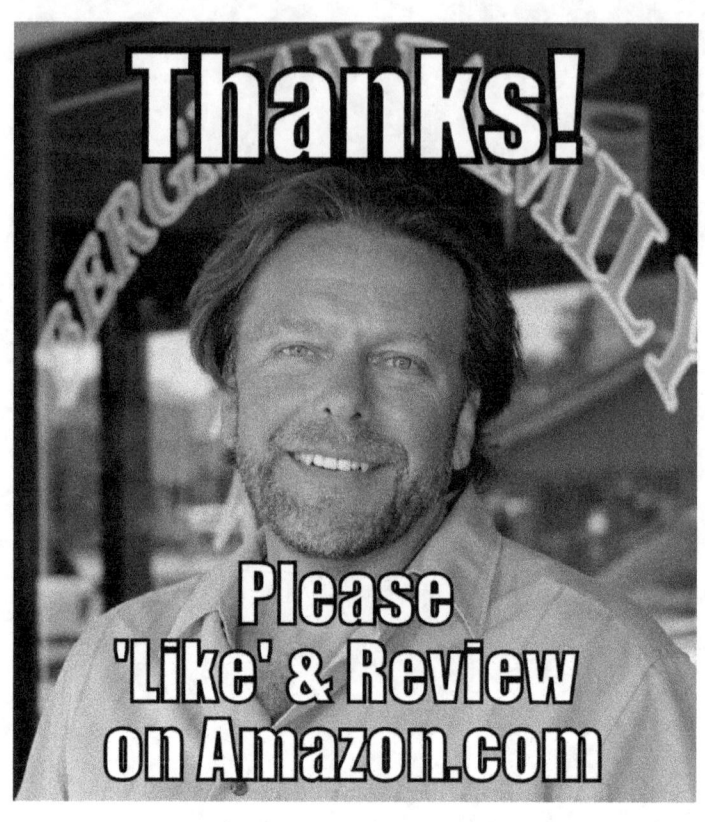

I you liked this book, you may be interested in some of the other books I have written.

How to Reverse Arthritis Naturally

How to Recover from Fibromyalgia: Real Solutions for a Real Problem

These books can be found in both Kindle and Paperback versions on Amazon.com.